# COMPLETE GUIDE TO GASTROENTERITIS

Comprehensive Strategies, Treatments, Prevention Tips, Your Essential Resource For Managing Stomach Infections, Diarrhea, And Vomiting

## DEHART HAIRSTON

© [DEHART HAIRSTON], [2024]

All rights reserved. No part of this publication may be reproduced, distributed, or transmitted in any form or by any means, including photocopying, recording, or other electronic or mechanical methods, without the prior written permission of the publisher, except in the case of brief quotations embodied in critical reviews and certain other noncommercial uses permitted by copyright law.

## DISCLAIMER

This book's content is only intended for general informative purposes. At the time of writing, the author has taken every precaution to guarantee that the material is correct and current. Nevertheless, the author disclaims all explicit and implicit representations and guarantees about the availability, appropriateness, correctness, completeness, and usefulness of the material on these pages.

Since the author is not a licensed medical practitioner, the material in this book shouldn't be interpreted as medical advice. Before making any modifications to their diet, exercise regimen, or medical treatment, readers are urged to speak with a licensed healthcare provider.

Moreover, the author has no connection to any of the businesses, organizations, or people that are discussed in this book. Any mentions of goods, services, businesses, or people are purely informative and do not indicate endorsement or suggestion.

This book's content is entirely dependent on the author's expertise, study, and comprehension of the topic. Despite having taken reasonable care to offer correct information, the author disclaims all liability for any mistakes or omissions in the material as well as for any losses, harm, or damages resulting from using the information.

It is recommended that readers use their own judgment and discretion when applying the knowledge in this book to their own situations. The use or implementation of any material in this book may result in unfavorable repercussions, directly or indirectly, for which the author assumes no liability.

By reading this book, you agree to release and hold the author harmless from any claims, losses, liabilities, costs, or expenditures resulting from or related to the use of the information you get from it.

## Table of Contents

### CHAPTER 1 ................................................................13
- **Introduction To Gastroenteritis**................................13
- **Understanding The Basics**......................................13
- **Causes And Symptoms**..........................................14
- **Importance Of Early Detection**...............................16

### CHAPTER 2 ................................................................19
- **How Gastroenteritis Spreads**..................................19
- **Routes Of Transmission**........................................19
- **Common Sources Of Infection**................................22
- **Preventive Measures**.............................................25

### CHAPTER 3 ................................................................29
- **Types Of Gastroenteritis**........................................29
- **Viral Gastroenteritis**..............................................29
- **Bacterial Gastroenteritis**........................................32
- **Parasitic Gastroenteritis**........................................35

### CHAPTER 4 ................................................................39
- **Diagnosing Gastroenteritis**....................................39
- **Medical History Assessment**..................................39
- **Physical Examination**............................................42
- **Laboratory Tests And Imaging**................................45

Laboratories Exams .................................................46
Imaging Research ...................................................47
## CHAPTER 5 ..................................................................51
Treatment Options ..................................................51
Fluid Replacement Therapy .....................................51
Dietary Recommendations ......................................54
Medications And Antidiarrheals ............................56
## CHAPTER 6 ..................................................................61
Managing Gastroenteritis In Children ...................61
Special Considerations For Pediatrics ..................61
Signs Of Dehydration .............................................64
Pediatric Treatment Guidelines .............................68
## CHAPTER 7 ..................................................................75
Preventive Strategies ..............................................75
Hand Hygiene Practices ..........................................75
Food Safety Tips .....................................................77
Vaccination Recommendations ..............................80
## CHAPTER 8 ..................................................................83
Complications And When To Seek Medical Help ..83
Recognizing Severe Symptoms ..............................83
Potential Complications ..........................................86

Emergency Warning Signs ............................................ 89

## CHAPTER 9 ................................................................ 93

Gastroenteritis In Special Populations ...................... 93

Elderly And Immunocompromised Individuals ..... 93

Pregnancy And Gastroenteritis ................................. 98

Travel-Related Concerns ........................................... 102

## CHAPTER 10 .............................................................. 107

Lifestyle Modifications For Prevention .................. 107

Building A Strong Immune System ........................ 107

Stress Management Techniques .............................. 109

Maintaining A Healthy Diet And Hydration Routine
....................................................................................... 112

CONCLUSION ............................................................ 115

THE END ...................................................................... 119

## ABOUT THIS BOOK:

"Gastroenteritis" is an essential resource for comprehending, averting, and controlling a prevalent gastrointestinal ailment that impacts individuals across the globe. This book is essential reading for anyone concerned with their health and well-being due to its extensive coverage of everything from fundamentals to advanced techniques.

In Chapter 1, readers are provided with an introductory overview of gastroenteritis, encompassing its causes, symptoms, and the critical significance of timely identification. By establishing the context for the subsequent content, the reader gains a comprehensive understanding of the condition.

Chapter 2 provides an in-depth analysis of the mechanisms by which gastroenteritis is transmitted, including common sources of infection and transmission routes. Readers who possess this information can adopt preventative measures to mitigate the likelihood of exposure.

In Chapter 3, an in-depth examination is conducted on the various classifications of gastroenteritis, encompassing parasitic, bacterial, and viral manifestations. This chapter provides readers with the necessary knowledge to discern and mitigate specific pathogens.

In Chapter 4, the diagnostic tools and techniques utilized to validate gastroenteritis are expounded upon, encompassing laboratory analyses, imaging, and medical history evaluations. This enables individuals to promptly seek medical attention and obtain suitable care.

Chapter 5 explores various treatment modalities, such as dietary supplements, fluid replacement therapy, and pharmaceutical interventions, providing readers with pragmatic approaches to symptom management and recovery promotion.

Chapter 6 delves into the management of gastroenteritis in children, with a particular focus on treatment guidelines and distinctive considerations that are specific to this patient population.

To conclude the book, chapters seven through ten offer readers invaluable perspectives on complications, preventive measures, lifestyle adjustments for prevention, and special populations. This comprehensive compilation of information guarantees that readers possess a well-rounded set of tools to safeguard their health.

Fundamentally, "Gastroenteritis" transcends its literary form and serves as a guide to wellness, providing readers with the information, resources, and tactics necessary to effectively manage and surmount this prevalent yet formidable ailment.

Whether one is a concerned parent, a healthcare professional, or an individual seeking to safeguard oneself and one's loved ones, this book is an essential and must-have resource.

# CHAPTER 1

## Introduction To Gastroenteritis

### Understanding The Basics

Gastroenteritis, also known as the stomach flu, is an intestinal and gastric inflammation-causing condition that impacts the gastrointestinal tract. Typical symptoms of this inflammation include nausea, vomiting, diarrhea, abdominal pain, and occasionally fever. In addition to viral, bacterial, and parasitic infections, specific medications, toxins, and food allergies may all contribute to its development.

The gastrointestinal tract is essential for nutrient absorption and digestion. Normal functioning is disrupted when it becomes inflamed as a result of gastroenteritis, which gives rise to the distinctive symptoms associated with the condition. Although gastroenteritis has the potential to impact individuals of all ages, it is notably prevalent among the elderly, young children, and those with compromised immune systems.

## Causes And Symptoms

Several distinct pathogens, such as bacteria, viruses, and parasites, are capable of inducing gastroenteritis. Viral gastroenteritis, commonly known as stomach flu, is a prevalent manifestation of the condition and is frequently induced by norovirus, rotavirus, and adenovirus, among others. Various bacteria, including Salmonella, Escherichia coli (E. coli), Campylobacter, and Shigella, can induce bacterial gastroenteritis. Conversely, parasitic gastroenteritis is predominantly caused by cryptosporidium and Giardia.

Symptoms of gastroenteritis may differ based on the underlying etiology of the infection and the general health status of the affected individual. Nevertheless, frequent manifestations encompass nausea, vomiting, diarrhea, abdominal cramping or pain, and occasionally, fever. The duration of these symptoms may exceed one week, spanning from a few days to several weeks, and may vary in intensity.

## Importance Of Early Detection

Detection of gastroenteritis as early as possible is critical for its effective management and treatment. Early detection of the symptoms can aid in the prevention of complications and the mitigation of the disease's severity. Symptoms such as persistent vomiting, diarrhea lasting for more than a few days, dehydration, high fever, severe abdominal pain, or blood in the stool should prompt you to seek medical attention.

While seeking medical attention, various measures can be implemented at home to alleviate the symptoms of gastroenteritis and facilitate the recovery process.

To prevent the spread of the infection, these include staying hydrated by consuming plenty of fluids, getting sufficient rest, avoiding foods that may irritate the stomach, and practicing good hygiene.

You can protect yourself and your loved ones from this occasional yet potentially fatal condition by acquiring a fundamental comprehension of gastroenteritis, including its causes, symptoms, and the criticality of early detection. Prompt medical intervention and diligent self-maintenance are essential for the successful treatment of the majority of gastroenteritis cases, enabling individuals to promptly resume their regular activities.

# CHAPTER 2

## How Gastroenteritis Spreads

### Routes Of Transmission

It is essential to comprehend the mode of gastroenteritis transmission to prevent its incidence and regulate its spread. Gastroenteritis, commonly known as the stomach flu, has the potential to propagate via diverse pathways, with the most common being contact with infected individuals, contaminated water, or food.

A principal mode of transmission involves the ingestion of food or water that has been contaminated. Food and water that are not handled, stored, or prepared with proper hygiene practices may become contaminated with bacteria, viruses, or parasites. For instance, water that originates from a contaminated source or food that is not cooked thoroughly may contain pathogens that induce gastroenteritis. Furthermore, the transmission of the illness can also occur via contact with contaminated surfaces or cross-contamination between raw and cooked foods.

Conversely, interpersonal contact serves as a prevalent mode of transmission. Germicidal pathogens are easily transmitted when an infected individual comes into contact with others, especially through proximity or the exchange of personal items. This may occur as a result of sharing utensils, shaking hands, or attending to a sick person without adhering to proper hygiene protocols.

Additionally, specific gastroenteritis-causing viruses, including norovirus, have the potential to disseminate via aerosolized particles in the atmosphere. Thus, if an individual who is infected expels virus-containing particles into the air via vomiting or diarrhea, those nearby may inhale them and thereby contract the infection.

A comprehensive comprehension of the diverse modes of transmission is imperative to efficiently execute preventive measures aimed at regulating the dissemination of gastroenteritis.

## Common Sources Of Infection

The identification of prevalent sources of infection is critical to mitigate the consequences of gastroenteritis outbreaks on communities and individuals. The proliferation of gastroenteritis-causing pathogens is facilitated by several factors, including contaminated food, water, and environmental surfaces.

A substantial source of infection for gastroenteritis is contaminated food. Salmonella, Escherichia coli (E. coli), Campylobacter, and other pathogenic bacteria that are present in raw or undercooked meats, poultry, seafood, and eggs, are capable of inducing gastrointestinal distress when ingested.

Norvirus and Giardia are two additional pathogens that can be transmitted through fruits and vegetables contaminated with feces during cultivation, harvesting, or processing.

Similarly, infected water presents a substantial hazard for the transmission of gastroenteritis. Ingestion of water from untreated or improperly treated sources, such as lakes, rivers, or wells, may result in the contamination of the water with pathogenic bacteria, viruses, or parasites. Substandard sanitation practices, including the inappropriate disposal of sewage or human waste, have the potential to introduce additional contaminants into water sources and exacerbate cases of gastroenteritis.

Environmental surfaces have the potential to act as reservoirs for gastroenteritis-causing infections. Contamination of shared objects and surfaces in public areas, including but not limited to doorknobs, handrails, and countertops, may occur as a result of contact with contaminated food or water or contact with infected individuals. Failure to adhere to appropriate hygiene protocols, including consistent handwashing and disinfection of surfaces, may result in the facilitation of the spread of agents that cause gastroenteritis among individuals.

By recognizing and mitigating these prevalent sources of infection, communities and individuals can adopt proactive strategies to safeguard against gastroenteritis and advance the welfare of the general public.

## Preventive Measures

To prevent gastroenteritis, a multifaceted strategy is required that addresses several transmission and infection control factors. The implementation of preventive measures can effectively mitigate the impact of gastroenteritis outbreaks on communities and individuals by reducing their frequency.

A highly effective preventive measure is the observance of good hygiene, specifically the application of appropriate handwashing techniques. By consistently cleansing hands with soap and water, particularly before meals, after restroom use, and after attending to an ill individual, one can effectively mitigate the transmission of pathogens that cause gastroenteritis. Thus, in situations where soap and water are not easily accessible, hand sanitizers containing a minimum of 60% alcohol may also be utilized as a substitute.

Additionally, it is critical to ensure the safety of food and water to prevent gastroenteritis. This entails cooking foods appropriately to eliminate bacteria, preventing the transfer of pathogens from raw to cooked foods, and limiting dairy product consumption to pasteurized options. It is recommended to consume bottled or boiled water while traveling or in regions with questionable water quality and to refrain from consuming ice produced from untreated water.

Implementing appropriate sanitation and disinfection protocols can additionally mitigate the likelihood of gastroenteritis transmission. This includes cleaning and disinfecting surfaces and objects that are frequently touched, such as electronic devices, doorknobs, and countertops. Furthermore, ensuring the timely and proper sanitary disposal of feces and sewage can contribute to the prevention of water source and environmental surface contamination.

In addition, individuals must observe proper food safety protocols during food preparation and handling. These include diligently washing hands and utensils, storing food at appropriate temperatures, and preventing cross-contamination between raw and cooked foods.

Through the consistent and effective implementation of these preventive measures, communities and individuals can mitigate the likelihood of contracting gastroenteritis and advance the general health and welfare of the public.

# CHAPTER 3

## Types Of Gastroenteritis

### Viral Gastroenteritis

Viral gastroenteritis, also referred to as viral stomach infection or stomach flu, is an exceptionally transmissible intestinal infection distinguished by inflammation of the intestines and stomach. Genoenteritis of this nature is predominantly induced by a variety of viruses, such as norovirus, rotavirus, adenovirus, and astrovirus.

Norvirus is a prevalent etiological agent of viral gastroenteritis, having caused epidemics in educational institutions, communities, and cruise ships across the globe.

Rapid transmission occurs via contaminated surfaces, food, water, and person-to-person contact. In contrast, infants and young children are primarily afflicted by rotavirus, which induces severe diarrhea and vomiting.

Typically manifesting between one and three days following viral exposure, viral gastroenteritis is characterized by nausea, vomiting, diarrhea, abdominal cramps, fever, headache, and muscle aches. Although the condition generally resolves on its own within a few days, it has the potential to cause dehydration, particularly in young children, older adults, and those with compromised immune systems.

The primary objectives of treatment for viral gastroenteritis are symptom relief and prevention of dehydration. This may entail consuming an adequate amount of fluids, such as oral rehydration solutions, to replenish depleted electrolytes and fluids. Hospitalization may be required for intravenous fluid administration in severe cases.

Adhering to proper hygiene practices is crucial in mitigating the transmission of viral gastroenteritis. This includes washing hands frequently with soap and water, particularly after using the restroom or changing diapers, and before food preparation or consumption. Furthermore, to mitigate the potential for transmission, it is advisable to disinfect contaminated surfaces and refrain from proximity to infected individuals.

## Bacterial Gastroenteritis

Bacterial gastroenteritis, alternatively referred to as bacterial food poisoning, manifests as an infection of the digestive tract caused by the contamination of food or water with pathogenic bacteria. Constraints regarding the bacterial causative agents of gastroenteritis comprise Salmonella, Campylobacter, Shigella, and Vibrio cholerae, all of which are prevalent.

Salmonella, a prevalent bacterium that causes bacterial gastroenteritis, is frequently linked to poultry, eggs, and unpasteurized dairy products that have been inadequately cooked. The spectrum of symptoms from mild to severe includes diarrhea, abdominal cramps, fever, nausea, and vomiting.

E. E. coli is a prevalent causative agent, wherein specific strains generate toxins that induce severe diarrhea, abdominal pain, and, in rare instances, hematochezia. This form of infection, named E. Escherichia coli O157:H7 has the potential to induce complications including hemolytic uremic syndrome (HUS), a critical renal disorder.

Bacterial gastroenteritis is treated by the pathogen type and severity of symptoms. Antibiotics are frequently prescribed to reduce the risk of complications and shorten the duration of illness.

Nevertheless, specific bacterial infections—such as those induced by particular strains of E. E. coli, which might defy antibiotic treatment, might instead necessitate supportive care.

Bacterial gastroenteritis can be prevented through the implementation of appropriate food handling and preparation protocols. These include ensuring that foods are cooked to their designated internal temperatures, preventing cross-contamination between raw and cooked foods, and promptly refrigerating perishable items. Additionally, it is critical to avoid consuming unpasteurized dairy products and contaminated water and to maintain proper hand hygiene.

## Parasitic Gastroenteritis

Parasitic gastroenteritis is caused by parasitic organisms, including Cyclospora, Giardia lamblia, Cryptosporidium, and Entamoeba histolytica, which infect the digestive tract. Typically, these parasites are transmitted via contact with infected animals or individuals, contaminated food, or water.

Cryptosporidium and Giardia lamblia are two prevalent parasitic species that are accountable for gastroenteritis on a global scale. Giardiasis, which is caused by Giardia lamblia, frequently results in weight loss, diarrhea, abdominal cramps, bloating, gas, and nausea. Aside from fever and vomiting, Cryptosporidiosis, which is caused by

Cryptosporidium, may also manifest with comparable symptoms.

An additional parasitic organism that can induce amoebic dysentery—a severe form of gastroenteritis distinguished by bloody diarrhea, abdominal pain, and fever—is Entamoeba histolytica. Although less prevalent in developed nations, it continues to be a substantial contributor to gastrointestinal ailments in areas where sanitation and hygiene standards are inadequate.

Medications designed to eradicate the parasite from the body, such as antiparasitic drugs like metronidazole or nitazoxanide, are commonly used to treat parasitic gastroenteritis. Prolonged support may be required alongside pharmacological intervention to mitigate symptoms and avert dehydration.

Safe drinking water practices, such as boiling or treating water from untreated sources, avoiding untreated water from lakes, rivers, or streams, and practicing good hygiene when traveling to regions with poor sanitation, are necessary to prevent parasitic gastroenteritis. In addition, the risk of parasitic infections can be reduced by avoiding raw or undercooked foods and by thoroughly washing fruits and vegetables before consumption.

38

# CHAPTER 4

## Diagnosing Gastroenteritis

### Medical History Assessment

In the process of diagnosing gastroenteritis, a comprehensive medical history is initially gathered. The healthcare provider conducts a comprehensive inquiry into the patient's medical history, current travel plans, dietary preferences, and any possible encounters with contagious diseases. The data acquired throughout this evaluation assists in ascertaining the probable etiology of gastroenteritis and provides direction for subsequent diagnostic inquiries.

Typically, patients are queried regarding the timing and duration of symptoms including dehydration, fever, diarrhea, vomiting, and abdominal pain. Also crucial are the severity of symptoms and any factors that may worsen or ameliorate them. Furthermore, the medical practitioner may request information regarding recent antibiotic usage, close contact with individuals who are ill, or ingestion of food or water that has been contaminated.

The occurrence of particular pathogens that cause gastroenteritis is more widespread in particular geographic areas, making travel history critical. Individuals who have recently undertaken international travel may have encountered distinct varieties of bacteria, viruses, or parasites that are uncommon in their country of origin.

Additionally, inquiries regarding pre-existing medical conditions, such as gastrointestinal disorders or immunocompromised status, may be incorporated into the medical history evaluation. These aspects are significant in determining the severity of gastroenteritis and its treatment. Additionally pertinent is the patient's medication history, which should include any recent substitutions or new prescriptions, given that specific medications may increase the risk of gastrointestinal symptoms.

In its entirety, a thorough evaluation of the patient's medical history yields significant knowledge regarding the potential cause of gastroenteritis, thereby informing subsequent diagnostic procedures and treatment determinations.

## Physical Examination

After reviewing the patient's medical history, a physical examination is performed to assess the patient's general well-being and identify any indications of gastroenteritis. Critical clinical findings that assist in confirming the diagnosis and quantifying the severity of the condition might be unveiled during this examination.

The healthcare provider conducts a vital signs assessment, which includes monitoring the patient's temperature, heart rate, blood pressure, and respiratory rate, to identify any indications of dehydration or systemic infection. Common complications of gastroenteritis include dehydration, which manifests as hypotension, tachycardia, and decreased skin turgor.

An abdominal examination may uncover symptoms such as distention, tenderness, or hyperactive bowel sounds, all of which are indicative of inflammation in the gastrointestinal tract and potentially signify gastroenteritis. By performing abdominal palpation, one can identify specific regions of discomfort and evaluate for indications of peritonitis or bowel obstruction, both of which may require additional diagnostic testing or intervention.

The healthcare provider may conduct a general physical examination, apart from evaluating the abdomen, to detect any additional indications of infection or systemic illness. An assessment of the skin, lymph nodes, and mucous membranes may yield information regarding the etiology of gastroenteritis or detect complications such as lymphadenopathy or cutaneous rashes.

In general, the physical examination holds significant importance in the diagnosis of gastroenteritis due to its ability to verify the existence of gastrointestinal symptoms, identify indications of dehydration or systemic infection, and guide subsequent diagnostic assessment and treatment.

## Laboratory Tests And Imaging

Imaging studies and laboratory tests are essential components in the diagnosis and treatment of gastroenteritis, especially when the cause is unknown or complications are suspected. These diagnostic modalities assist in the identification of the fundamental etiology of gastroenteritis, evaluation of potential complications, and guidance of suitable treatment approaches.

**Laboratories Exams**

1. Stool analysis involves the collection and examination of stool samples to detect the presence of pathogenic microorganisms, including bacteria, viruses, and parasites. To identify particular pathogens, microscopy, culture, and polymerase chain reaction (PCR) analysis are frequently employed techniques.

2. **Blood Tests:** To detect indications of dehydration, electrolyte imbalances, or systemic infection, blood tests may be performed. Complete blood count (CBC), electrolyte levels, renal function tests, and inflammatory markers including C-reactive protein (CRP) and erythrocyte

sedimentation rate (ESR) are typical laboratory parameters that are assessed.

**3. Additional Laboratory Tests:** By the clinical presentation and presumed cause, further laboratory investigations may be warranted. These may include antigen detection assays, serological tests targeting particular pathogens, or assessments for inflammatory markers linked to specific gastrointestinal disorders.

Imaging Research

**1. Abdominal X-ray:** To detect indications of bowel obstruction, perforation, or other structural irregularities, an abdominal X-ray may be obtained. This imaging modality can detect gastroenteritis complications that necessitate immediate intervention.

**2. Ultrasound of the Abdomen:** An ultrasound of the abdomen may be performed to evaluate the gastrointestinal tract for signs of inflammation, fluid accumulation, or other abnormalities. The utilization of this non-invasive imaging modality can yield significant insights regarding the magnitude and gravity of complications associated with gastroenteritis.

**3. Computed Tomography (CT) Scan:** A CT scan of the abdomen may be recommended to assess for complications including abscess formation, perforation, or ischemic bowel disease in cases of severe or complicated gastroenteritis. CT imaging provides visualization of abdominal structures in high resolution and, if necessary, can aid in guiding surgical treatment.

In general, laboratory tests and imaging studies are significant instruments in the diagnostic process of gastroenteritis, as they empower medical practitioners to ascertain the fundamental etiology, evaluate potential complications, and customize therapeutic strategies according to the unique requirements of each patient. The utilization of these diagnostic modalities is of the utmost importance in enhancing patient outcomes and mitigating the potential for chronic complications linked to gastroenteritis.

# CHAPTER 5

## Treatment Options

### Fluid Replacement Therapy

Fluid replacement therapy is an essential component of gastroenteritis treatment, with the dual objectives of averting dehydration and reinstating electrolyte homeostasis. Violent and diarrhea-induced fluid and electrolyte loss during gastroenteritis can rapidly result in dehydration if adequate replenishment is not administered. Dehydration has the potential to worsen symptoms and give rise to severe complications, particularly among susceptible demographics such as elderly individuals and young children.

The principal objective of fluid replacement therapy is to efficiently restore depleted electrolytes and fluids. Oral rehydration solutions (ORS) are frequently employed to treat gastroenteritis of mild to moderate severity. These solutions comprise electrolytes such as sodium and potassium, along with a precise proportion of sugar and water, which aid in replenishing lost fluids and preserving the electrolyte equilibrium of the body. Because it is easily administered and readily available over the counter, ORS is an excellent option for at-home treatment.

In patients with gastroenteritis who are unable to tolerate oral fluids or who have more severe cases of the disease, intravenous (IV) fluid therapy may be required. This process entails the intravenous administration of fluids and electrolytes into the bloodstream. IV fluid therapy is commonly administered under the supervision of healthcare professionals in a hospital or clinic environment. It facilitates swift rehydration and is especially advantageous for those who are unable to retain fluids as a result of persistent vomiting.

During gastroenteritis, fluid intake must be closely monitored, particularly in children and the elderly, who are at a greater risk of dehydration. Dry mouth, sunk eyes, decreased urine output, lethargy, and irritability are all indicators of dehydration. If you or a family member encounter these symptoms, it is imperative that you seek immediate medical attention.

## Dietary Recommendations

The management of one's diet is of paramount importance in the management of gastroenteritis, as it serves to mitigate symptoms, facilitate recovery, and avert additional inflammation of the gastrointestinal tract. Equally as important as staying hydrated during gastroenteritis is selecting nutritious foods to alleviate symptoms and promote healing.

When symptoms such as vomiting and diarrhea are at their most severe during the acute phase of gastroenteritis, it is best to consume a bland, easily digestible diet that will not irritate the stomach and intestines. Bananas, rice, applesauce, toast (BRAT diet), plain crackers, boiled potatoes, and boiled chicken are examples of such foods. These palatable foods have the potential to promote bowel regularity and alleviate diarrhea.

Progressively reintegrate additional food items into your dietary regimen as your symptoms subside and your appetite resurfaces. Begin with digestible alternatives such as cooked vegetables, lean proteins, and whole grains. Fatty, highly seasoned, or spicy foods should be avoided, as they can cause digestive irritation and worsen symptoms.

In addition to selecting nutritious foods, it is critical to be mindful of your eating technique. By consuming frequent, small meals throughout the day, one can mitigate symptoms such as nausea and bloating and prevent the digestive system from becoming overloaded. To facilitate digestion, ensure that you chew your food thoroughly and eat slowly.

## Medications And Antidiarrheals

Medication may occasionally be prescribed to treat gastroenteritis symptoms and accelerate recovery. Nevertheless, exercising prudence is imperative when ingesting medications, particularly over-the-counter (OTC) alternatives, because their efficacy may vary among individuals and may occasionally exacerbate symptoms or disrupt concurrent therapies.

Antidiarrheal medications, including bismuth subsalicylate (Pepto-Bismol) and loperamide (Imodium), are frequently employed to manage diarrhea and decrease the frequency of bowel movements. These pharmaceutical agents function by impeding intestinal motility, thereby facilitating the absorption of water and electrolytes and leading to the formation of more compact bowel movements.

Although antidiarrheal medications have the potential to alleviate diarrhea, their efficacy varies among individuals.

Certain medical conditions, such as inflammatory bowel disease or infectious diarrhea caused by specific bacteria or parasites, should be approached with caution when using these substances. Doing so may potentially prolong the illness or result in complications. Before using antidiarrheal medications, it is vital to consult a healthcare professional, particularly if you have preexisting conditions or are currently taking other medications.

Other medications may be prescribed in addition to antidiarrheals to treat specific symptoms of gastroenteritis, including antiemetics for the management of nausea and vomiting and antibiotics to combat bacterial infections.

Nevertheless, antibiotics are generally prescribed only in the treatment of bacterial gastroenteritis and are ineffective against parasitic or viral infections.

When taking medications for gastroenteritis, adhere to your healthcare provider's instructions at all times, and never exceed the recommended dosage. It is strongly advised to promptly seek medical attention if any adverse reactions or symptoms worsen while taking medications.

# CHAPTER 6

## Managing Gastroenteritis In Children

## Special Considerations For Pediatrics

Children with gastroenteritis necessitate particular care owing to their diminutive stature and distinct physiological requirements. In contrast to adults, children exhibit elevated metabolic rates, rendering precipitous and suitable management imperative due to their susceptibility to dehydration. In addition, children may have a diminished capacity to articulate their symptoms in the same manner as adults, which can complicate the process of diagnosis and treatment.

When pediatric gastroenteritis occurs, the risk of dehydration is a critical factor to consider. Young children, particularly infants and toddlers, have reduced fluid reserves that render them more vulnerable to dehydration. Rapid dehydration has the potential to give rise to severe complications if not promptly attended to. Consequently, in children with gastroenteritis, parents and caregivers should be vigilant in their observation for indicators of dehydration.

Additionally, the possibility of electrolyte imbalances in children with gastroenteritis is a crucial factor to consider. Electrolytes, including sodium, potassium, and chloride, are essential for cellular and organ function and fluid homeostasis. Prolonged episodes of vomiting and diarrhea that are linked to gastroenteritis have the potential to cause substantial electrolyte losses, which can exacerbate dehydration and give rise to complications including metabolic acidosis.

Moreover, there may be variations in the etiology of gastroenteritis between minors and adults. Although rotavirus and norovirus are prevalent viral pathogens that can cause gastroenteritis in children and adults, bacterial and parasitic infections may be more prevalent in pediatric cases. The differentiation holds significance due to its potential impact on treatment choices, including the administration of antiparasitic or antibiotic drugs.

In brief, the management of gastroenteritis in children necessitates distinct approaches owing to their unique physiological characteristics, elevated susceptibility to dehydration, and possible variations in etiology in comparison to adults. Accurate identification of symptoms, diligent observation for dehydration, and suitable intervention are critical in pediatric patients to guarantee optimal results.

## Signs Of Dehydration

To effectively treat gastroenteritis, it is critical to recognize the symptoms of dehydration, especially in children who are more susceptible to fluid loss.

Dehydration manifests when the body expends excess fluids relative to what it consumes, resulting in electrolyte imbalances that have the potential to induce severe health complications. Diarrhea and vomiting are symptoms of gastroenteritis that can complicate the process of fluid loss, thereby elevating the risk of dehydration considerably.

Increased desire is an early indicator of dehydration in infants. Children might exhibit heightened thirst or request beverages more frequently than customary. Furthermore, dehydration may be indicated by parched or adhesive mucous membranes, including lips that are chapped or a dry mouth. Reduced mucus production during sobbing may also indicate depletion in neonates.

As the condition of dehydration advances, additional symptoms may manifest. These may manifest as reduced fluid consumption leading to concentrated urine, as evidenced by decreased urine output or darker urine. Additionally, children may exhibit signs of lethargy or irritability, as well as a loss of interest in play or other activities and diminished energy. Additionally, severe cases of dehydration may manifest as sunken eyes and a sunken fontanelle, which is the tender area located on the cranium of a neonate.

Changes in the turgor of the epidermis may also serve as an indicator of dehydration. The capacity of the skin to revert to its original position following a pinprick or draw is referred to as skin turgor. The epidermis of dehydrated children may exhibit reduced elasticity and a delayed restoration to its typical condition. This can be determined by observing the rate of return to normal after gently compressing the skin on the back of the hand or abdomen.

In general, prompt identification of the indicators of dehydration is critical for effective management of gastroenteritis. Parents and caregivers must exercise caution in monitoring for indications of dehydration, including but not limited to increased thirst, decreased urine output, behavioral changes, and alterations in skin turgor. If these symptoms manifest, they should promptly seek medical attention.

## Pediatric Treatment Guidelines

It is of the utmost importance to adhere to pediatric treatment guidelines when managing gastroenteritis in children to maximize outcomes and minimize the likelihood of complications. Treatment guidelines serve as a set of evidence-based recommendations that healthcare providers can rely on when it comes to the management of gastroenteritis in pediatric patients.

These guidelines provide direction on matters such as fluid resuscitation, nutritional support, and medication administration.

Oral rehydration therapy is a fundamental component of treatment guidelines for gastroenteritis in pediatric patients. Oral rehydration therapy (ORT) entails the administration of solutions that precisely balance glucose and electrolytes to replenish fluids and electrolytes that have been lost due to diarrhea and vomiting. These solutions can aid in the prevention or correction of dehydration in children with gastroenteritis and are readily assimilated by the body.

When pediatric guidelines identify mild to moderate dehydration, ORT is frequently the initial treatment of choice. It is advisable to motivate children to consume oral rehydration solution in frequent, small doses to avoid gastric overload and enhance absorption. It is imperative to provide parental and caregiver education regarding the appropriate methods of preparing and administering oral rehydration solutions, as well as guidance on how to observe for indications of improvement or decline.

Intravenous (IV) rehydration may be required in infants who are unable to tolerate oral fluids or in more severe cases of dehydration. IV rehydration enables prompt correction of electrolyte imbalances and dehydration through the direct administration of fluids and electrolytes into the circulation. It is crucial for healthcare providers to diligently observe children undergoing intravenous rehydration for indications of electrolyte imbalances or fluid excess.

Furthermore, pediatric treatment guidelines may encompass suggestions regarding the control of particular symptoms or complications that are linked to gastroenteritis. Antiemetic medications, for instance, may be prescribed to ameliorate nausea and vomiting, whereas antimotility compounds may, in certain instances, be utilized to reduce diarrhea. Nonetheless, clinical evaluation should guide the prudent and prudent use of these medications to prevent potential adverse effects.

In addition, nutritional support is a critical component of pediatric gastroenteritis treatment guidelines. A decrease in appetite and consumption of solid foods may occur in children who have gastroenteritis, which can result in nutritional deficiencies and worsen dehydration. As tolerated, medical professionals may advise a progressive reintegration into a standard diet, commencing with inodorous, readily digestible foods like toast, bananas, and rice.

In general, strict adherence to pediatric treatment guidelines is critical for the efficient management of pediatric gastroenteritis. Healthcare practitioners can enhance outcomes and mitigate the likelihood of complications in pediatric patients with gastroenteritis by adhering to evidence-based guidelines concerning oral rehydration, fluid resuscitation, nutritional support, and symptom management.

# CHAPTER 7

## Preventive Strategies

### Hand Hygiene Practices

Ensuring consistent hand hygiene is critical for mitigating the transmission of gastroenteritis. Hands serve as conduits through which pathogenic bacteria and viruses are transmitted; therefore, practicing proper hand hygiene can substantially mitigate the likelihood of acquiring and disseminating gastroenteritis.

It is of the utmost importance to consistently cleanse your hands with soap and water, particularly after using the lavatory, before food preparation or consumption, and after handling potentially contaminated items. Hand hygiene entails performing a minimum 20-second cleansing motion with detergent, paying particular attention to the areas between fingertips, beneath fingernails, and the backs of the hands.

When detergent and water are not easily accessible, alcohol-based hand sanitizers can be utilized as a viable substitute. It is imperative to verify that the hand sanitizer comprises a minimum of 60% alcohol and scrub it meticulously across all finger surfaces until dried.

It is also vital to avoid contacting your face with unhygienic hands, particularly your mouth, nostrils, and eyes.

Mitigating exposure to these mucous membranes, which serve as entry points for pathogens, can substantially diminish the likelihood of infection.

Furthermore, promote the adoption of proper hand hygiene practices among your family, colleagues, and acquaintances, as well as those in your immediate vicinity. You can mitigate the transmission of gastroenteritis and foster a healthier environment by employing these practices collectively.

## Food Safety Tips

Foodborne gastroenteritis is frequently caused by ingesting contaminated foods or beverages; therefore, it is vital to practice proper food preparation and management. One can reduce the likelihood of contracting gastrointestinal distress and imbibing harmful pathogens by adhering to food safety guidelines.

Before handling food, begin by ensuring that your hands and cooking surfaces are spotless. To prevent cross-contamination, wash fruits and vegetables thoroughly under running water and use separate cutting surfaces for uncooked meat, poultry, seafood, and produce.

Ensure that food reaches the proper internal temperature before heading to eliminate any microorganisms that may be present. Verify that meats, poultry, fish, and leftovers are prepared to the recommended temperatures using a food thermometer. To inhibit the development of pathogens, perishable foods should be promptly refrigerated.

It is advisable to refrain from ingesting unpasteurized dairy products and raw or undercooked meats, as these may contain pathogenic bacteria including Salmonella, E. coli as well as Campylobacter. Furthermore, exercise prudence when dining out, especially at establishments where food handling procedures or hygiene practices are dubious.

To prevent the accumulation of pathogens, clean and sanitize kitchen surfaces, utensils, and appliances regularly. Particular focus should be directed toward surfaces that are in direct contact with uncooked foods, including refrigerator handles, cutting boards, and countertops.

One can ensure the enjoyment of meals without concern for the occurrence of contaminated gastroenteritis by strictly adhering to these food safety guidelines.

## Vaccination Recommendations

A critical factor in the prevention of specific strains of gastroenteritis, especially those caused by viral pathogens like rotavirus and norovirus, is vaccination. Vaccines elicit the production of antibodies by stimulating the immune system, thereby conferring immunity against distinct viral strains and mitigating the intensity of symptoms in the event of infection.

Routine vaccination against rotavirus is advised for neonates and young children by the standard immunization schedule. Vaccination against Rotavirus, which is the primary cause of severe diarrhea and dehydration in neonates and young children across the globe, can substantially mitigate the disease burden.

Those who are more susceptible to norovirus infection, including healthcare workers, travelers, and residents of communal environments, may also derive advantages from accessible vaccines, in conjunction with rotavirus vaccination. At present, no vaccine is authorized for norovirus; however, continuous research endeavors are focused on the development of efficacious vaccines to avert this exceptionally transmissible gastrointestinal ailment.

It is advisable to seek guidance from your healthcare provider to ascertain the recommended vaccines for you and your family, taking into consideration factors such as age, medical history, and risk factors. You can strengthen your body's defenses against gastroenteritis and contribute to community-wide efforts to contain its transmission by maintaining current vaccinations.

# CHAPTER 8

## Complications And When To Seek Medical Help

### Recognizing Severe Symptoms

Recognizing severe symptoms is critical in the context of gastroenteritis to ensure prompt intervention and management. Although spontaneous resolution is commonplace within a few days, specific symptoms may suggest the presence of a more severe underlying condition or complication. Knowing these symptoms enables individuals to promptly seek medical assistance.

Severe gastroenteritis is characterized by chronic or extreme dehydration. Dehydration is characterized by excessive fluid loss beyond the body's intake, resulting in the impairment of vital physiological processes. Excessive thirst, parched mouth, decreased urine output, dark-colored urine, fatigue, vertigo, and confusion are all symptoms of dehydration. Observe infants and young children for the following symptoms: drooping eyes, absence of fluid production during periods of weeping, and prolonged dry diaper usage.

An additional cause for concern is the detection of blood in bowel movements or regurgitation. Vomit that is bloody may have a coffee grounds-like consistency or a vibrant red hue, both of which are indicative of upper gastrointestinal tract hemorrhage. Fecal blood may take the form of red streaks, maroon-colored feces, or black, tarry feces, all of which indicate hemorrhage originating from the lower gastrointestinal tract. Both situations necessitate prompt medical attention to ascertain the underlying cause and commence suitable treatment.

Moreover, the presence of intense abdominal pain coupled with a fever may indicate a more critical bacterial or parasitic infection. Although fever is a physiological reaction to an underlying infection, the presence of extremely high temperatures, coupled with severe abdominal pain, ought to indicate the need for medical attention. Furthermore, if symptoms endure for an extended period without exhibiting signs of amelioration or if there is a significant deterioration in general well-being, a medical assessment is necessary to exclude the possibility of complications and guarantee appropriate therapeutic intervention.

## Potential Complications

Although complications are uncommon in cases of gastroenteritis, specific factors may increase the risk of developing more severe complications. It is critical to comprehend these potential complications to promptly identify and intervene.

Dehydration is a notable complication that has the potential to progress swiftly, especially among susceptible populations including neonates, young children, elderly adults, and those with compromised immune systems. If left untreated, severe dehydration may result in complications such as kidney dysfunction, electrolyte imbalances, and shock. Oral or intravenous rehydration therapy is essential for the management of dehydration and the prevention of further complications.

Beriatric or parasitic infections represent an additional possible complication. Pathogenic bacteria, including Campylobacter, Salmonella, or Escherichia coli (E. coli), as well as parasitic organisms such as Giardia or Cryptosporidium, can occasionally induce gastroenteritis. If not appropriately managed, these infections have the potential to result in more severe symptoms, an extended duration of illness, and systemic complications. It may be imperative to administer antibiotics or antiparasitic drugs to eliminate the pathogen and avert potential complications.

Seldom, especially in patients with compromised immune systems, can gastroenteritis result in systemic infections or sepsis. When the body's response to an infection induces systemic inflammation, sepsis may ensue, which has the potential to result in organ dysfunction and eventual failure. Antimicrobial therapy and supportive care must be administered promptly to prevent further deterioration and improve prognoses.

## Emergency Warning Signs

Specific indicators that prompt urgent medical intervention are present in cases of gastroenteritis. It is critical to not disregard these emergency warning signs, as they could indicate critical complications that may be fatal and necessitate immediate intervention.

A persistent and unyielding sensation of severe abdominal pain or discomfort is one such indicator. Although gastroenteritis frequently causes abdominal distress, the presence of severe or localized pain could potentially signify a more critical underlying condition, including appendicitis, intestinal obstruction, or perforation.

Immediately seek medical attention if the pain is severe or if it is accompanied by other worrisome symptoms.

Additionally, altered mental status, bewilderment, or lethargy are severe indicators. Severe dehydration, electrolyte imbalances, or systemic infection are all conditions that may be indicated by these neurological symptoms and necessitate prompt medical evaluation and intervention. Mental status changes should always be taken seriously and warrant an immediate visit to the emergency department for comprehensive evaluation and treatment.

In addition, symptoms such as respiratory difficulties, rapid pulse rate, or episodes of dizziness necessitate immediate medical intervention. Systemic complications, such as sepsis or electrolyte imbalances, which have the potential to disrupt critical organ function, could be indicated by these symptoms. It is critical to intervene immediately to stabilize the patient and avert additional deterioration.

It is critical to recognize severe symptoms, comprehend potential complications, and observe emergency warning signs to effectively manage gastroenteritis.

Prompt medical intervention has the potential to alleviate complications, enhance prognoses, and guarantee a complete recuperation. Always seek prompt medical advice when in doubt to address any concerns and obtain the appropriate care.

# CHAPTER 9

## Gastroenteritis In Special Populations

## Elderly And Immunocompromised Individuals

**Comprehension of Vulnerabilities**

Regarding gastroenteritis, the elderly and those with compromised immune systems encounter particular obstacles. The immune system's resistance to pathogens may be compromised due to age-related alterations in the digestive system, rendering the geriatric more vulnerable to infections. In a similar vein, individuals with compromised immune systems, such as those who are chemotherapy-treated or who have HIV/AIDS, experience a reduced capacity to combat infections, including gastroenteritis.

**Recognizing Symptoms**

It can be difficult to diagnose gastroenteritis in these populations because symptoms may manifest otherwise or be obscured by underlying conditions. Although healthy individuals frequently experience diarrhea, vomiting, and abdominal discomfort, the elderly may manifest more nuanced symptoms including perplexity, lethargy, or exacerbation of pre-existing conditions. Individuals with compromised immune systems may also manifest more severe symptoms or endure longer durations of illness.

## The Criticality of Timely Treatment

To prevent complications, elderly and immunocompromised patients require immediate treatment. Dehydration poses a substantial risk, particularly among the elderly, and failure to promptly address it may result in severe health complications. Treatment strategies may require modification in light of factors such as the patient's age, pre-existing medical conditions, and immune system. Potential strategies to effectively manage symptoms include administering intravenous fluids, altering medication dosages, or providing supplementary support.

## Preventive Actions

In these susceptible populations, gastroenteritis prevention requires a combination of hygienic practices and, where applicable, vaccination. Hand hygiene should be emphasized by caregivers, particularly before handling food or attending to the needs of the elderly or those with compromised immune systems. Additionally, the risk of transmission can be reduced by avoiding contact with contaminated surfaces and infected individuals. Certain healthcare providers may advise against the use of vaccines, such as the influenza vaccine, to protect against specific strains of gastroenteritis.

## Assistance and Monitoring

Providing supportive care and monitoring are critical components in the management of gastroenteritis among immunocompromised elderly patients. Consistent monitoring of vital signs, electrolyte levels, and hydration status can aid in the early detection of complications. Caregivers must verify that the individual is hydrated and obtaining sufficient nutrition to facilitate their recuperation. When complications develop or in severe cases, hospitalization may be required to facilitate specialized treatment and closer monitoring.

# Pregnancy And Gastroenteritis

## Particular Considerations

Gastroenteritis that occurs during pregnancy gives rise to unique complications owing to the potential hazards it poses to the unborn child and the expectant mother. Hormonal fluctuations that impact the digestive tract and immune system may prolong the severity of gastroenteritis symptoms in pregnant women. Moreover, the adverse effects of vomiting and diarrhea-induced dehydration on the health of both the mother and the fetus are significant.

## Safely Managing Symptoms

Aside from the well-being of the expectant mother, healthcare providers must prioritize the safety of the fetus when treating gastroenteritis in pregnant women. Anti-diarrheal and antiemetics, which are frequently prescribed for symptom management, may not be contraindicated during pregnancy on account of potential adverse effects on the developing embryo. However, treatment frequently centers around implementing supportive measures such as rest, hydration, and dietary adjustments.

## The Monitoring of Difficulties

Gastroenteritis during pregnancy necessitates vigilant observation to detect dehydration and other potential complications that may compromise the health of both the mother and fetus. Routine check-ups may be advised by healthcare providers to evaluate the fetus's health, electrolyte levels, and hydration status. A hospital stay may be required in extreme circumstances to administer intravenous fluids and to ensure that both the mother and the embryo are closely monitored.

**Preventive Measures**

Pregnant women can prevent gastroenteritis by adhering to proper sanitation practices and refraining from known sources of infection. It is advised that pregnant women engage in regular hand hygiene practices, particularly before handling or ingesting food, and refrain from proximity to individuals who are ill. In addition to maintaining adequate hydration, consuming safe, well-prepared foods can aid in preventing gastroenteritis during pregnancy.

**Obtaining Medical Care**

Pregnant women who develop symptoms of gastroenteritis must seek immediate medical attention to protect the health of both the mother and the fetus. Healthcare professionals possess the ability to evaluate the intensity of symptoms, prescribe suitable therapeutic interventions, and oversee for possible complications. Pregnant women must engage in candid communication with their healthcare providers regarding any symptoms or concerns they may be experiencing.

## Travel-Related Concerns

### Travel-Related Gastroenteritis Dangers

A variety of environmental factors and pathogens that are encountered during travel can elevate the susceptibility to gastroenteritis. Travel-associated gastroenteritis can be triggered by contamination with novel or resistant strains of bacteria or viruses, alterations in water quality, and modifications in weight. The presence of frequent symptoms such as fever, diarrhea, vomiting, and abdominal pain can cause significant inconvenience and disrupt travel arrangements.

**Preventive Measures**

The prevention of gastroenteritis associated with travel begins with meticulous preparation and planning. As well as researching destination-specific health hazards, such as the stability of food and water, tourists should take the necessary precautions. This may entail refraining from consuming fresh or undercooked foods, potable water, and ice, in addition to practicing proper hand hygiene and employing alcohol-based hand sanitizers in situations where detergent and water are unavailable.

**Asphyxiation and Vaccination**

Preventing particular strains of gastroenteritis may require the administration of prophylactic medications or vaccinations in certain instances. Vaccines targeting prevalent pathogens that may be encountered during travel to specific regions can offer protection against diseases including cholera, typhoid fever, and hepatitis A. In addition, prophylactic antimicrobial therapy may be advised for individuals at high risk or those embarking on journeys to regions where resistance to common antibiotics is well-documented.

**Medical Attention Abroad**

It is critical to seek medical attention immediately if gastroenteritis develops while traveling, particularly if symptoms are severe or persistent. If necessary, appropriate treatment may be administered at local healthcare facilities and may consist of rehydration therapy, antiemetics, and antimicrobial medications. Additionally, pertinent insurance information and medical records should be accessible to travelers to facilitate treatment while they are abroad.

**Post-Travel Remainder**

Those who have returned from a trip with gastroenteritis should closely monitor their symptoms and seek medical attention if they persist or deteriorate. Post-travel medical evaluation may be required in certain circumstances to exclude the possibility of complications or persistent infections. Informing healthcare providers about any ailments contracted during travel can facilitate the provision of suitable follow-up treatment and mitigate the risk of infection transmission.

# CHAPTER 10

## Lifestyle Modifications For Prevention

## Building A Strong Immune System

A strong immune system is the body's first line of defense against gastroenteritis and a host of other illnesses. It's like having an army ready to drive out intruders at any time. But how can we reinforce this essential protection system?

Sleep should be your priority. Sleep is when most of your body's healing process takes place. Try to get between seven and nine hours of good sleep every night to help your immune system recover. Exercise regularly is also essential. Exercise improves circulation, which makes it possible for immune cells to move freely throughout the body and carry out their function. A little workout or even just a strenuous stroll might have a big impact.

Additionally, make sure you're getting enough minerals and vitamins. Whole grains, lean meats, fruits, and vegetables are nutrient-rich meals that provide your immune system with the fundamental components it needs to operate at its best. Consider taking supplements containing immune-supporting vitamins such as zinc, vitamin D, and C if your diet isn't providing enough.

Finally, never undervalue the importance of relaxing. Prolonged stress weakens the immune system, increasing your vulnerability to illnesses like gastroenteritis. Include stress-relieving activities in your everyday routine, such as deep breathing exercises, meditation, or enjoyable hobbies. By maintaining your mental health, you're strengthening your body's defenses against illness.

## Stress Management Techniques

Tension has become an inevitable part of life for many people in today's fast-paced society. But long-term stress may wreak havoc on your body, especially your digestive system. Effective stress management is crucial to avoiding gastroenteritis and preserving general health.

Mindfulness meditation is one of the best methods for managing stress. By focusing on the here and now and noticing your thoughts and feelings without passing judgment, you may cultivate mindfulness. Frequent meditation has been shown to improve temperament, lower stress levels, and increase general well-being. Practicing mindfulness meditation for even a short period each day may significantly lower your stress levels.

Progressive muscle relaxation is another useful method. Starting from your ankles and working your way up to your head, you will tense and then slowly release every muscle group in your body. Progressive muscular relaxation may promote calmness and relaxation while easing physical strain.

Deep breathing techniques may also aid in lowering tension and triggering the body's relaxation response. Try inhaling slowly and deeply through your nose, filling your lungs, and then slowly and deliberately exhaling through your mouth. Repeat this numerous times, paying attention to the way your breath enters and leaves your body each time.

Last, but not least, it might be helpful to find constructive ways to release stress, such as doing things you like, going outside, or talking to loved ones. You may lessen your chance of developing gastroenteritis and shield your digestive system from the damaging effects of ongoing stress by adopting these stress management practices into your daily routine.

## Maintaining A Healthy Diet And Hydration Routine

What you put into your body affects not just how susceptible you are to gastroenteritis but also your general state of health. Maintaining the healthiest possible functioning of your gastrointestinal system and preventing infections requires a well-balanced diet high in nutrients and water.

Firstly, make sure you are well hydrated. Every cell, tissue, and organ in your body—including the gastrointestinal tract—needs water to operate properly. Try to drink eight 8-ounce glasses of water or more if you're active or in a humid atmosphere each day. If regular water doesn't appeal to you, consider adding some taste by infusing it with citrus such as cucumber or lemon.

Focus on including a variety of nutrient-dense items in your diet when it comes to eating. This includes an abundance of fruits and vegetables, which are rich in antioxidants, vitamins, and minerals that support the immune system and general health. To complete your meals and provide you with energy for the whole day, choose lean meats, whole grains, and healthy fats.

Another crucial element of a balanced diet is fiber, especially for gastrointestinal health.

Fiber promotes the growth of healthy intestinal flora, controls digestion, and keeps people from becoming constipated. Make a point of eating a wide variety of foods high in fiber, such as fruits, vegetables, whole grains, legumes, and seeds.

Lastly, watch how much alcohol and caffeine you consume. Both may cause the body to become dehydrated, which may impede digestive processes and raise your chance of developing gastroenteritis. Reduce your intake of alcohol and stimulants and replace them with hydrating drinks like coconut water, herbal tea, or water.

You can provide your body with the vital nutrients and fluids it needs to perform at its best and guard against gastroenteritis and other gastrointestinal problems by adhering to a balanced diet and hydration regimen.

## CONCLUSION

In summary, gastrointestinal tract inflammation is the hallmark of gastroenteritis, a common and often self-limiting illness. Gastritis is usually brought on by bacterial or viral infections, but it may also be brought on by parasites, toxins, or even certain drugs. Its symptoms may vary from mild to severe and include vomiting, diarrhea, fever, and stomach discomfort. In certain instances, these symptoms can cause dehydration and electrolyte abnormalities.

Supportive therapy, which includes appropriate hydration, electrolyte restoration, and symptomatic relief, is the main emphasis of gastroenteritis management. Most of the time, the illness clears itself in a few days without the need for specialized medical care. But in susceptible groups including young children, the elderly, and those with weakened immune systems, gastroenteritis may present serious health concerns and may need medical intervention to avoid complications.

Taking preventive action is essential for lowering the prevalence and spread of gastroenteritis. The risk of infection may be reduced by using safe food handling procedures, immunizing against certain microorganisms, and practicing good hand hygiene. The transmission of the illness may also be prevented by keeping a clean environment and avoiding contact with infected objects or people.

Although gastroenteritis usually resolves on its own, in high-risk cases, it may lead to consequences such as electrolyte imbalances, dehydration, and subsequent infections. For the illness to be properly managed, timely symptom assessment, early action, and appropriate medical treatment are thus crucial.

In conclusion, gastroenteritis is a frequent gastrointestinal illness that may have a range of etiologies, signs, and consequences. The effect of gastroenteritis on people and communities may be reduced by taking preventative measures, managing the illness promptly, and providing supportive care, all of which will enhance the quality of life and health outcomes.

**THE END**

www.ingramcontent.com/pod-product-compliance
Lightning Source LLC
Chambersburg PA
CBHW070259230526
45470CB00002B/648